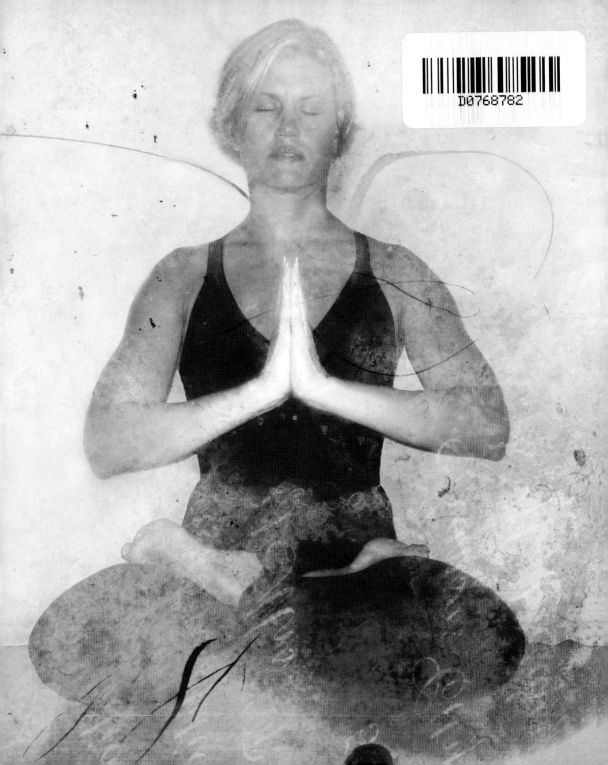

Effort and Surrender

The Art and Wisdom of Yoga

Effort and Surrender

The Art and Wisdom of Yoga

EDITED AND ILLUSTRATED BY
ERIC DINYER

FOREWORD BY
CAROLYN HOWARD-JOHNSON

AFTERWORD BY
MAX STROM

Andrews McMeel
Publishing

Kansas City

04 05 06 07 08 WKT 10 9 8 7 6 5 4 3 2 1

ISBN: 0-7407-4690-1

LIBRARY OF CONGRESS CONTROL NUMBER: 2004102678

ART DIRECTION: CRAIG NEUMAN

YOGA POSES: GRETCHEN ROBINSON

ATTENTION: SCHOOLS AND BUSINESSES

ANDREWS MCMEEL BOOKS ARE AVAILABLE AT QUANTITY DISCOUNTS WITH BULK PURCHASE FOR EDUCATIONAL, BUSINESS, OR SALES PROMOTIONAL USE. FOR INFORMATION, PLEASE WRITE TO: SPECIAL SALES DEPARTMENT, ANDREWS MCMEEL PUBLISHING, 4520 MAIN STREET, KANSAS CITY, MISSOURI 64111.

THE MYSTICISM OF YOGA IS THIS: THAT WE CAN STEP
UP TO OUR MAT—AND TO OUR LIVES—WITHOUT
EXPECTATION OF HOW THINGS WILL TURN OUT, AND
WITH THAT, FINALLY BEGIN TO EXPERIENCE OURSELVES
AS WE TRULY ARE: LIGHT, SPONTANEOUS, RESILIENT,
STRONG AND SUPPLE IN SPIRIT, AND FULLY OPEN TO
EACH MOMENT OF GRACE AS IT COMES.
THAT IS THE PRACTICE OF YOGA.

———— DOUG KELLER

Foreword

By Carolyn Howard-Johnson

Yoga is life. We see its splendor if we look,
know its challenges when we choose to, know
its comforts when we acknowledge them.
We recognize pain as a companion
from whom we can learn or turn away.
It can quiet like the curve
of an egg in a bowl.
It can be personal as a pulse
or connect like a current.
Life. We select its ecstasies.

I have been doing yoga since my brother directed me
in a few poses. I lay on a delicate patterned
Oriental carpet before a fire in my mother's home;
he pointed my limbs in the proper directions.
"Hatha Yoga," my brother said, "just poses."
I did "poses only" until I saw light and knew.
That was my only lesson.

My yoga instructor did not believe that yoga should be uncomfortable or difficult, but joyful. "Ignore those who say 'No pain, no gain,'" he said. "Stretch until it feels good. Breathe until it feels better."

Some poses came naturally. I have long muscles with little structure. Working them is like stretching warm Play-Doh. Poses like the Plow that are difficult for some were easy for me. At sixty-three I still do that extension with variations, knees touching the floor above my head. Some poses impart balance, like the Airplane Pose. My ability to do them improved as I practiced, mostly without my perceiving the changes because yoga benefits deliberately, leisurely. Some, like the Crane Posture, require strength. I do not expect ever to achieve them.

HAVING SAID THAT, IT DOES NOT MATTER TO ME. YOGA IS
NOT A CONTEST WITH OTHERS NOR WITH MYSELF.

IF PRACTICED, IT WILL PROGRESS. I DID NOT TAKE
EXPENSIVE LESSONS, USE SPECIAL EQUIPMENT, BUY A ZEN
WARDROBE, OR EVEN SET GOALS. ALL ONE NEEDS FOR
YOGA IS WILLINGNESS.

YOGA SIMPLY IS.

LIKE LIFE.

LIKE LOVE.

WHEN WE DO IT WE MAY ALSO CONNECT.

ERIC DINYER'S ETHEREAL PHOTOGRAPHS, AGED LIKE A
SIENNA LANDSCAPE AND COUPLED WITH QUOTES OF
SPIRITUAL ENCOURAGEMENT, COULD EASILY BE THE ROUTE
A BEGINNER OR A YOGA SAGE MIGHT TAKE TO THE NEXT
STEP. SUCH INSPIRATION WILL SURELY MOVE THE READER
TOWARD EFFORT AND SURRENDER. THE YOGA IS IN THE
DOING. YOGA, VERY SIMPLY, IS LIFE.

(EDITOR'S NOTE: CAROLYN HOWARD-JOHNSON IS THE AWARD-WINNING
AUTHOR OF *This Is the Place* AND *Harkening: A Collection of Stories Remembered*.
SHE IS AN INSTRUCTOR WITH UCLA'S WRITER'S PROGRAM AND HAS
BEEN A PRACTITIONER OF YOGA FOR THIRTY YEARS.)

*Y*OUR BODY, AND NOT ANY EDIFICE
BUILT BY HUMAN HANDS,
IS YOUR LIVING TEMPLE.
ENTER THE INNER SILENCE, AND
WORSHIP THERE.
SEND RAYS OF DEVOTION IN
SOLEMN PROCESSION UP THE
AISLE OF THE SPINE FROM YOUR
HEART TO THE HIGH ALTAR IN
THE FOREHEAD, THE SEAT OF
SUPERCONSCIOUS ECSTASY.

———— J. DONALD WALTERS
(SWAMI KRIYANANDA)

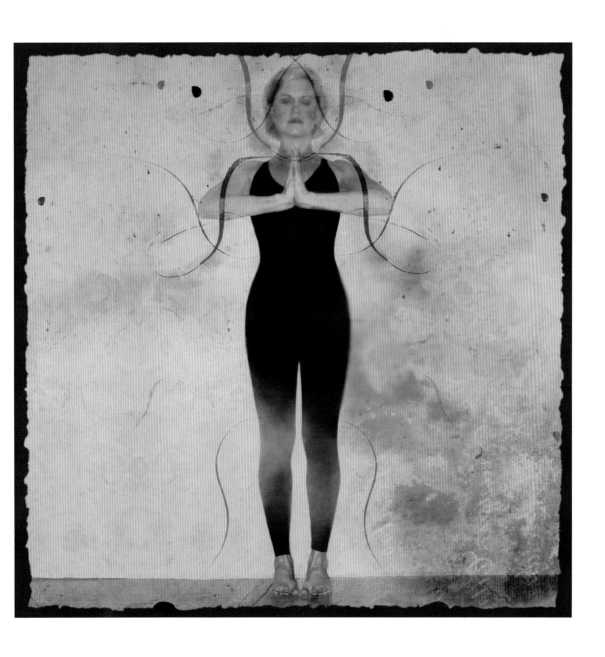

Mountain Pose: Tadasana

SHAKE THE CONTAINER AND THE CONTENTS SPILL. MOVE THE BODY AND THE MIND LOSES CONCENTRATION. FORCE THE BODY TO STAY STILL AND IT REBELS. TEACH THE BODY TO SURRENDER, RELAX YOUR MUSCLES AND NERVES, LET GO OF THEM FROM YOUR MIND: THE MIND BECOMES FREE OF THE BONDAGE OF THE FLESH. THIS IS THE SURRENDER OF THE BODY TO THE MIND, AND THE MIND WILL CONTINUE TO TAKE CARE OF THE BODY WITHOUT CATERING TO ITS EVERY WHIM.

——————— PANDIT USHARBUDH ARYA

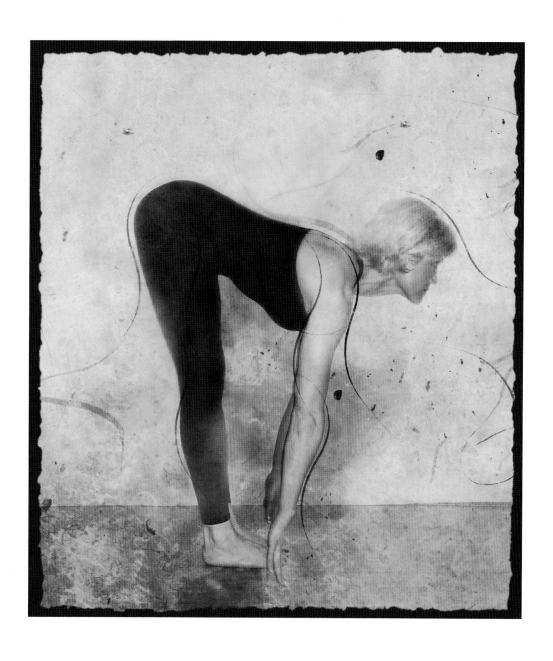

Uttanasana with Head Up: Urdhva Mukha Uttanasana

*M*ALE AND FEMALE, LIGHT AND SHADOW, EFFORT AND SURRENDER ARE SOME OF THE COMMON DUALITIES THAT EXIST IN OUR WORLD. ONE OF THE FIRST PRINCIPLES WE DISCOVER IN YOGA IS THE DYNAMIC PLAY OF OPPOSITES IN THE PRACTICE OF EACH ASANA. THROUGH YOGA WE LEARN HOW TO INTEGRATE OPPOSITES AND FIND THE BALANCE POINT BETWEEN THE BODY AND THE MIND.

——— JOHN FRIEND

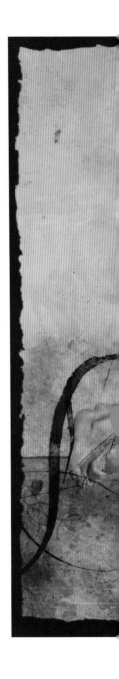

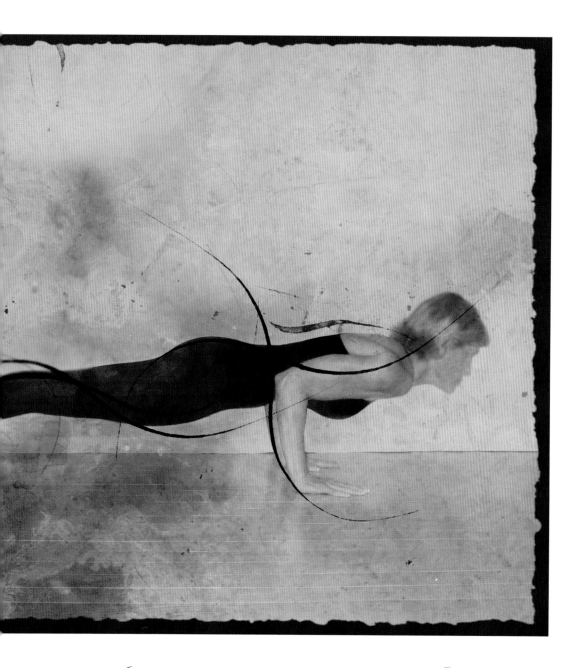

Four-Limbed Staff Pose: Chaturanga Dandasana

*T*HE PURPOSE OF YOGA IS TO
DEVELOP THE BODY, DISCIPLINE
THE MIND, AND STABILIZE THE
EMOTIONS IN ORDER TO REFINE
US AS A WHOLE.

———— B. K. S. IYENGAR

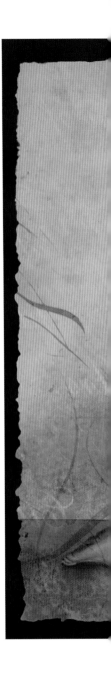

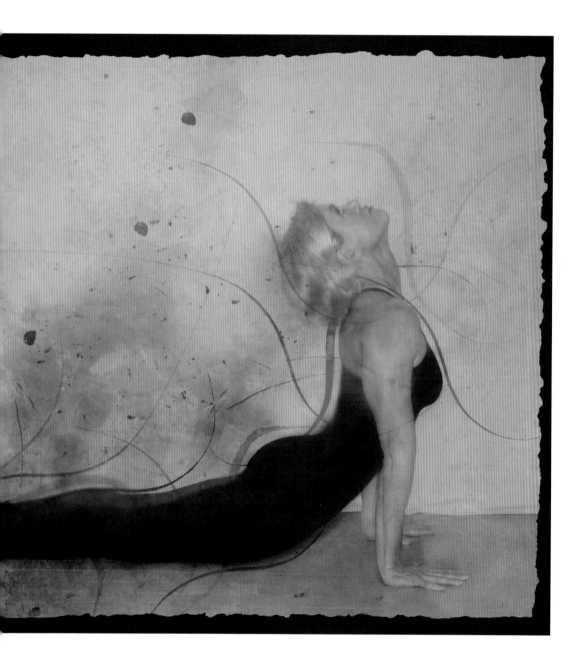

Upward-Facing Dog: Urdhva Mukha Svanasana

𝒯O PRACTICE YOGA IN
THE DEEPEST SENSE IS TO
COMMIT TO DEVELOPING
AWARENESS BY OBSERVING OUR
LIVES: OUR THOUGHTS, OUR
WORDS, AND OUR ACTIONS.

—————JUDITH LASATER, PH.D., P.T.

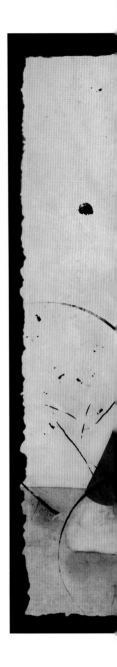

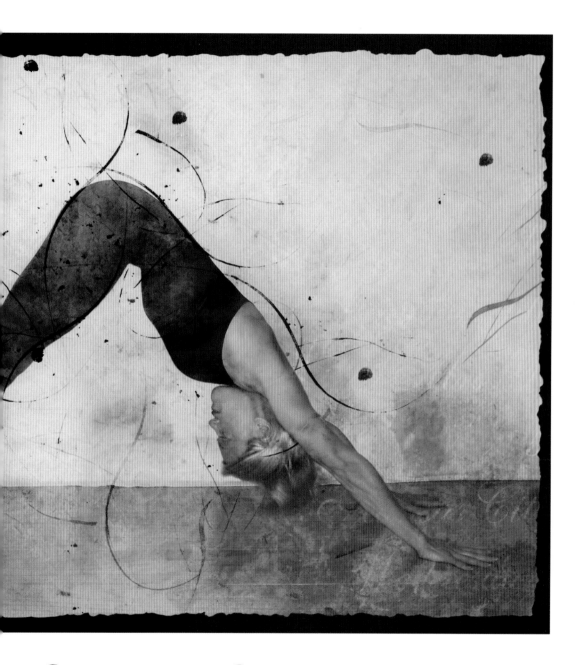

Downward-Facing Dog: Adho Mukha Svanasana

*I*N THIS VERY BREATH THAT WE
TAKE NOW LIES THE SECRET
THAT ALL GREAT TEACHERS TRY
TO TELL US.

——— PETER MATTHIESSEN

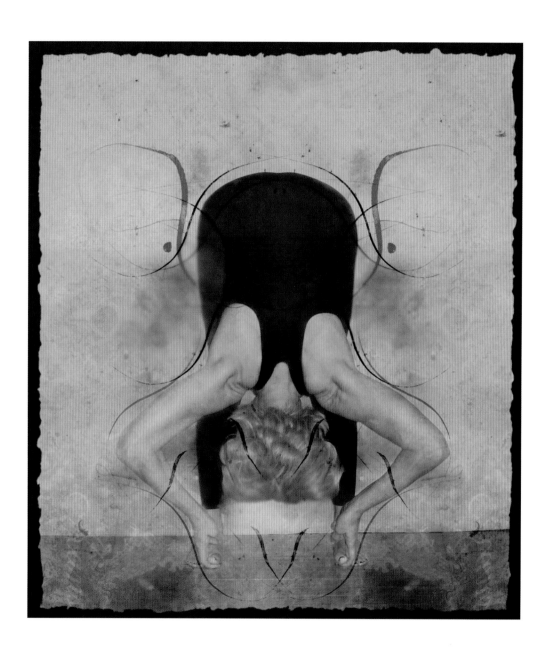

Foot Big Toe Pose: Padangusthasana

DO NOT FIGHT YOUR BODY.
DO NOT CARRY THE WORLD ON
YOUR SHOULDERS LIKE ATLAS.
DROP THE HEAVY LOAD OF
UNNECESSARY BAGGAGE AND YOU
WILL FEEL BETTER.
DO NOT KILL THE INSTINCT OF
THE BODY FOR THE GLORY OF
THE POSE. DO NOT LOOK AT
YOUR BODY LIKE A STRANGER,
BUT ADOPT A FRIENDLY APPROACH
TOWARD IT. WATCH IT, LISTEN TO
IT, OBSERVE ITS NEEDS, ITS
REQUESTS, AND EVEN HAVE FUN.
PLAY WITH IT AS CHILDREN DO;
SOMETIMES IT BECOMES VERY
ALERT AND SWIFT.
TO BE SENSITIVE IS TO BE ALIVE.

——— SWAMI KARMANANDA SARASWATI

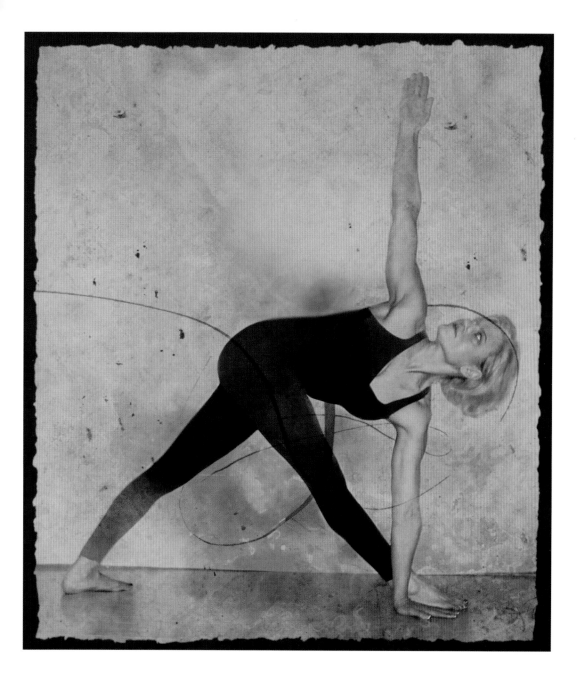

Triangle Pose: Trikonasana

PAIN IS YOUR BEST FRIEND.
IT IS INFINITELY MORE HONEST
WITH YOU THAN PLEASURE.
DESPITE WHAT YOU MIGHT THINK,
THE PAINFUL EXPERIENCES YOU
HAVE HAD BENEFIT YOU FAR
MORE THAN THE PLEASURABLE
ONES, EVEN THOUGH MOST OF US
SPEND OUR LIVES TRYING TO
DUCK AND HIDE FROM THEM.
BUT WHEN YOU CAN CENTER
YOURSELF AND BE OPEN TO LOOK
PAIN DEAD IN THE EYE, THEN
YOU HAVE TRANSCENDED THE
LIMITS OF YOUR EGO AND THIS
HUMANITY. IT IS THEN THAT YOU
ENTER INTO THE POSSIBILITY OF
BECOMING A GREAT BEING.

———— SWAMI CHETANANANDA

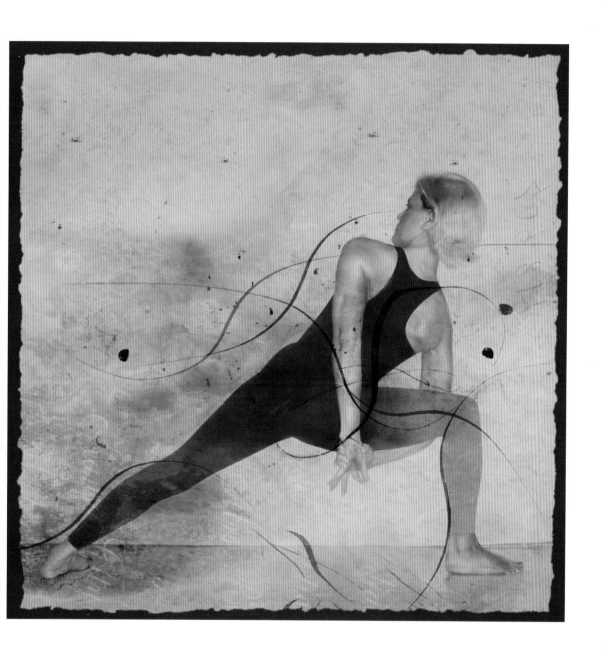

Extended Side Angle with Wrap: Utthita Parsvakonasana

THE BODY IS MY TEMPLE AND
ASANAS ARE MY PRAYERS.

WHILE PRACTICING ASANAS,
LEARN THE ART OF ADJUSTMENT.

WHEN YOUR POSTURE IS
IMBALANCED, THE PRACTICE
IS PHYSICAL; BALANCED ASANAS
LEAD TO SPIRITUAL PRACTICE.

———— B. K. S. IYENGAR

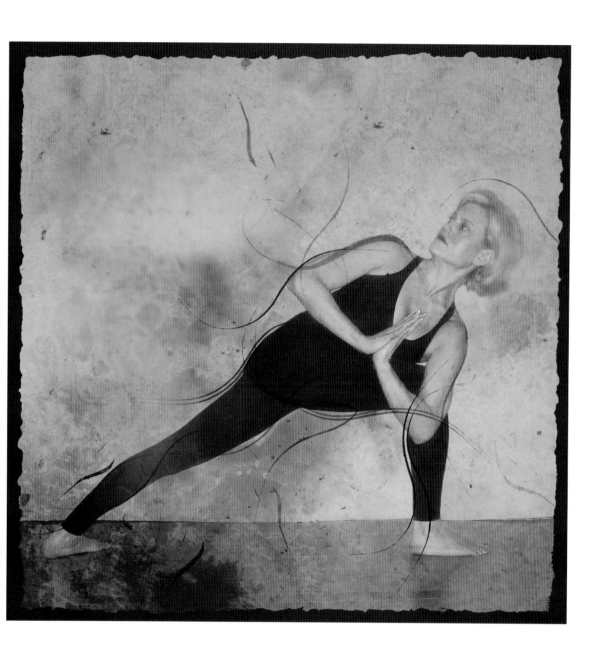

Prayer Twist: Parivritta Parsvakonasana

STAY PRESENT TO YOUR BODILY SENSATIONS. IF YOU TRY TO PULL SURRENDER TO YOU OR PUSH DISCOMFORT AWAY, YOU WILL CREATE EVEN MORE AGITATION. ENGAGE LIFE BY ACCEPTING THE SENSATIONS AS THEY ARE. AS YOU CONTINUE, YOU MAY NOTICE THAT YOU BEGIN TO RELAX AND THAT YOUR MIND IS NOT GRIPPED SO TIGHTLY AROUND THE OUTCOME.

——— JUDITH LASATER, PH.D., P.T.

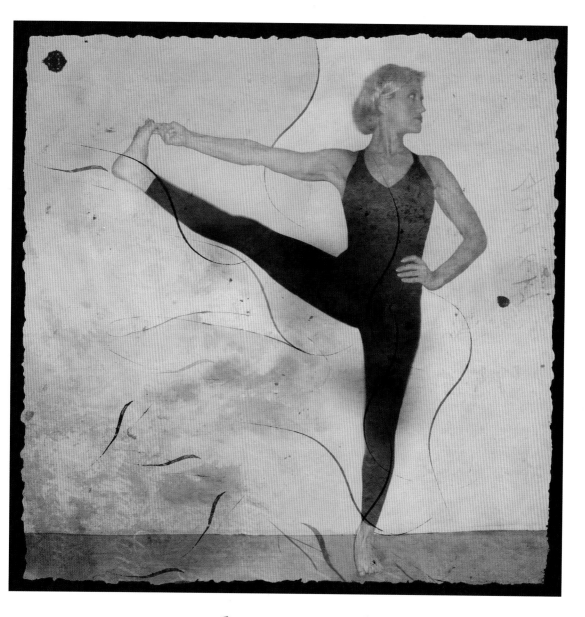

Extended Hand to Big Toe Posture:
Utthita Hasta Padangusthasana

*Y*OU MUST BE FIRMLY ROOTED.
SUCH IS THE FIRST LAW. THEN
GROW AND ASSERT YOURSELF.
AT THIS MOMENT OPEN
YOURSELF, STRETCH OUT YOUR
ARMS TO FEEL YOUR RADIATION
AROUND YOU, AND THEN BRING
THE UNIVERSE BACK TO YOU
WITH YOUR HEAD HELD HIGH,
FOR IT TOUCHES THE SUN.
BE DEEP, WIDE, TALL, TRULY A
TREE OF LIFE.

—————— LIZELLE REYMOND

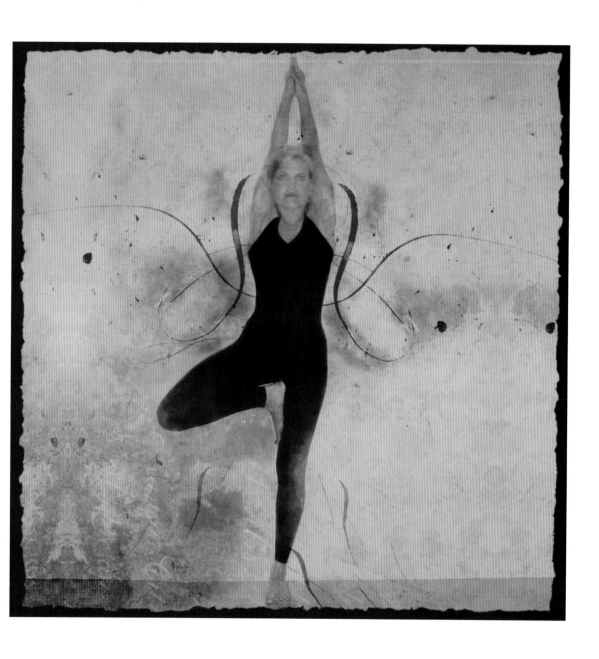

Tree Pose: Vrksasana

THE BODY IS LIKE AN AIRPLANE, INSIDE WHICH IS SEATED THE PILOT AND SELF, CAPTAIN AND MASTER. MINDSTUFF IS LIKE THE ENGINE OF THE AIRPLANE, AND SENSES ARE LIKE WINGS. BY MEANS OF THIS AIRPLANE OF BODY AND MIND, SELF FLIES PEACEFULLY AND CAREFULLY OVER MOUNTAINS, RIVERS, AND VALLEYS OF PROBLEMS.

———— RAMMURTI S. MISHRA

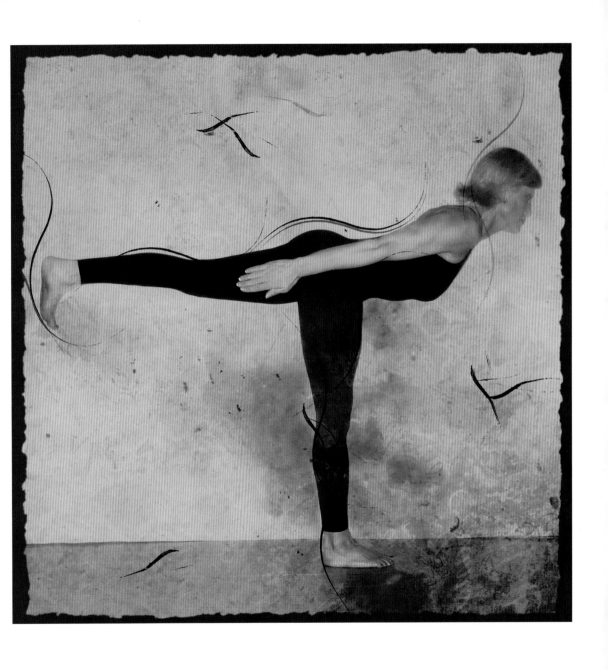

Airplane Posture: Virabhadrasana C

*Y*OGA IS A WAY OF MOVING INTO STILLNESS IN ORDER TO EXPERIENCE THE TRUTH OF WHO YOU ARE.

——— ERICH SCHIFFMANN

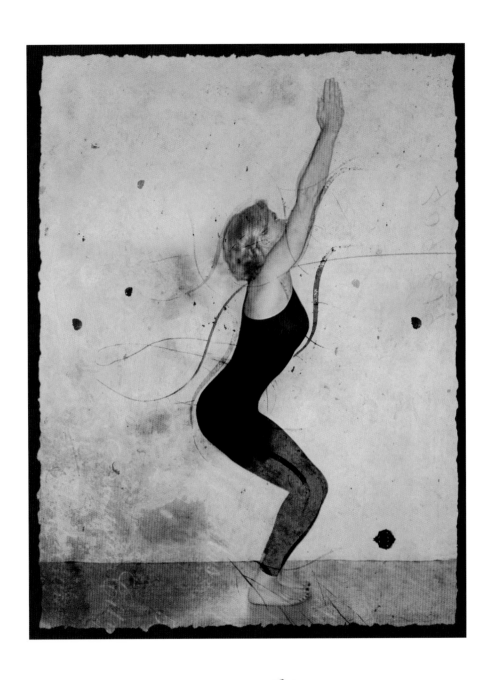

Chair Posture: Utkatasana

THE BREATH IS ONE OF THE BEST
MEANS FOR OBSERVING YOURSELF
IN YOUR YOGA PRACTICE.
HOW DOES THE BODY RESPOND
TO THE BREATH AND HOW DOES
THE BREATH RESPOND TO THE
MOVEMENT OF THE BODY?
THE BREATH SHOULD BE
YOUR TEACHER.

——— T. K. V. DESIKACHAR

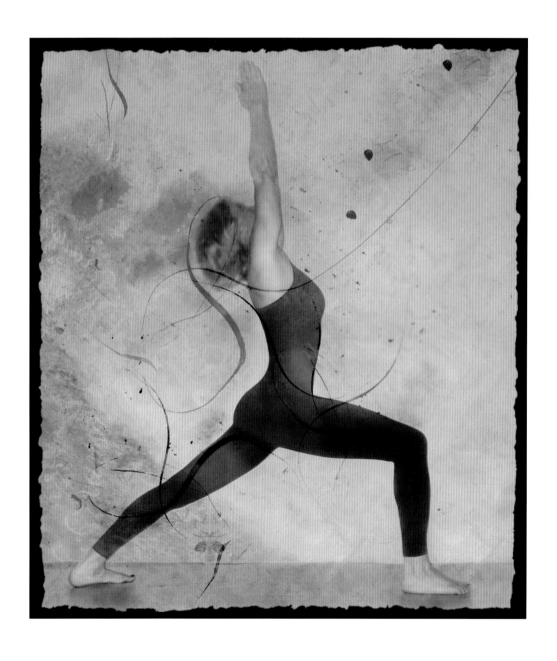

Warrior I: Virabhadrasana A

REMEMBER, YOGA PRACTICE IS LIKE AN OBSTACLE RACE: MANY OBSTRUCTIONS ARE PURPOSELY PUT IN THE WAY FOR US TO PASS THROUGH. THEY ARE THERE TO MAKE US UNDERSTAND AND EXPRESS OUR OWN CAPACITIES. WE ALL HAVE THAT STRENGTH, BUT WE DON'T SEEM TO KNOW IT. WE SEEM TO NEED TO BE CHALLENGED AND TESTED IN ORDER TO UNDERSTAND OUR OWN CAPACITIES. IN FACT, THAT IS THE NATURAL LAW. IF A RIVER JUST FLOWS EASILY, THE WATER IN THE RIVER DOES NOT EXPRESS ITS POWER. BUT ONCE YOU PUT AN OBSTACLE IN THE FLOW BY CONSTRUCTING A DAM, THEN YOU CAN SEE ITS STRENGTH IN THE FORM OF TREMENDOUS ELECTRICAL POWER.

———— SWAMI SATCHIDANANDA

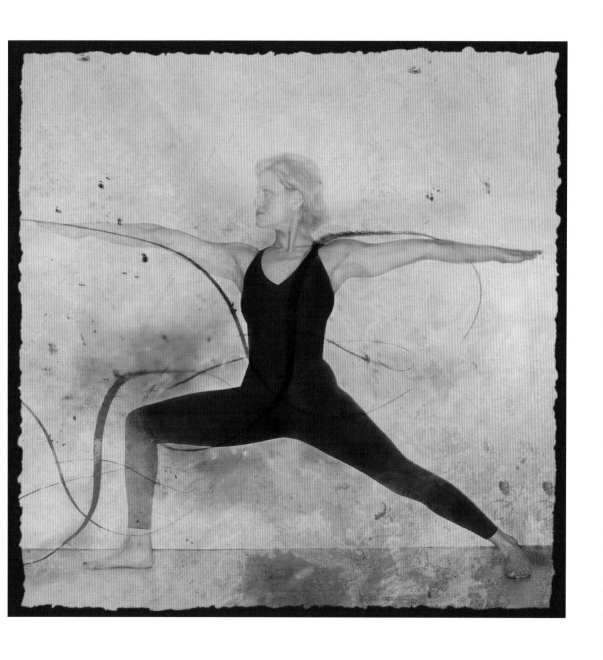

Warrior II: Virabhadrasana B

THE ART OF REVEALING
BEAUTY LIES IN REMOVING
WHAT CONCEALS IT.

———— JUDITH LASATER, PH.D., P.T.

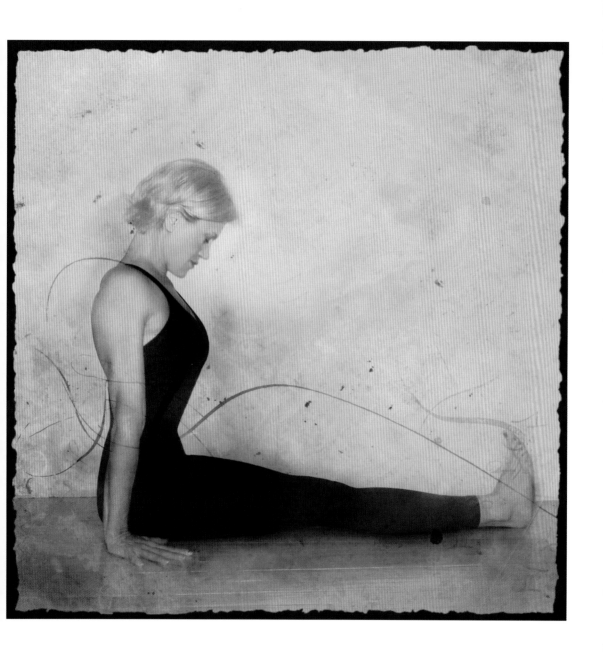

Staff Posture: Dandasana

OUR BREATH IS CONSTANTLY
RISING AND FALLING, EBBING
AND FLOWING, ENTERING AND
LEAVING OUR BODIES.
FULL BODY BREATHING IS AN
EXTRAORDINARY SYMPHONY OF
BOTH POWERFUL AND SUBTLE
MOVEMENTS THAT MASSAGE OUR
INTERNAL ORGANS, OSCILLATE
OUR JOINTS, AND ALTERNATELY
TONE AND RELEASE ALL THE
MUSCLES IN THE BODY. IT IS A
FULL PARTICIPATION WITH LIFE.

———— DONNA FARHI

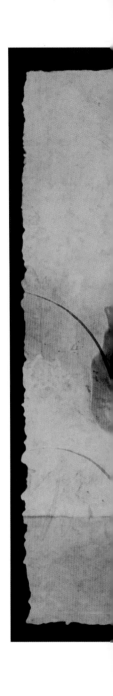

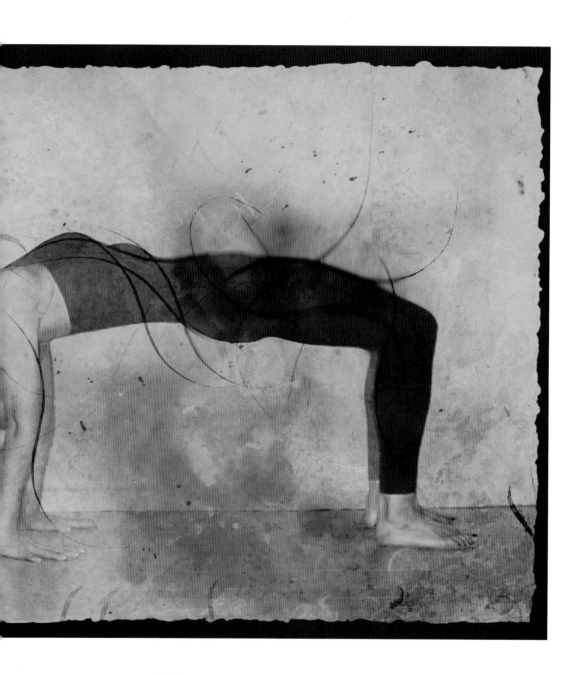

Table Posture: Purvottanasana

*Y*OGA IS A VISUAL ART,

SINCE THE BODY IS MADE TO

FORM GEOMETRICAL DESIGNS,

LINES, ARCHITECTURAL SHAPES,

AND THE LIKE, WHICH ARE

BEAUTIFUL TO BEHOLD.

——— B. K. S. IYENGAR

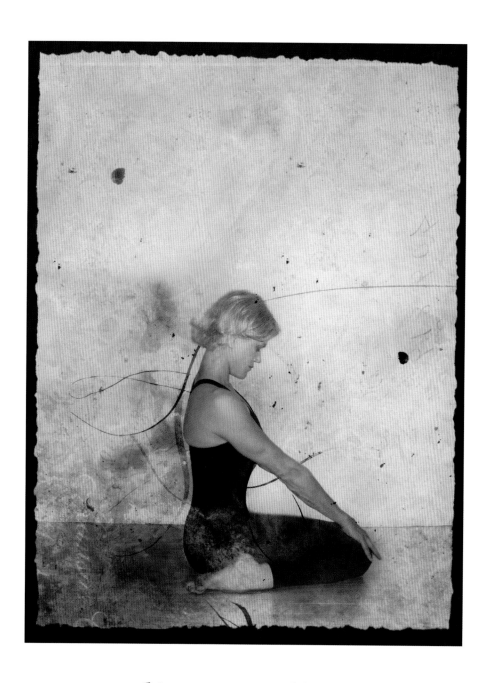

Hero's Posture: Virasana

*I*N A WORLD OF IMAGE MAKERS
PUTTING A "SPIN" ON FACTS,
YOGA TAKES A STAND FOR
THE AUTHENTIC AND
THE ETERNAL.

———— VICTORIA MORAN

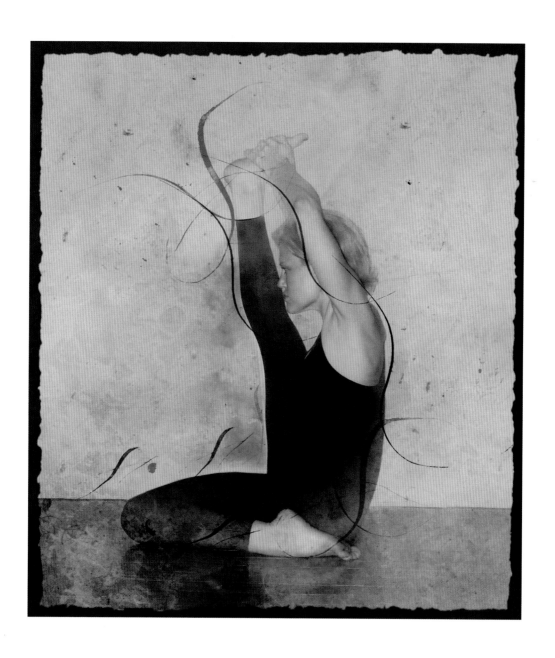

Heron Pose: Krounchasana

*W*HEN THE PRACTICE OF POSTURES IS COMBINED WITH CONSCIOUS BREATHING AND DEEP STATES OF CONCENTRATION AND ABSORPTION, PRANA (LIFE FORCE) WILL SOMETIMES SPONTANEOUSLY "TAKE OVER" THE PRACTICE. SUDDENLY, ENERGY ITSELF WILL BEGIN TO DIRECT THE FLOW OF POSTURES. IN THESE MOMENTS WE MAY HAVE A SENSE OF EFFORTLESSNESS, OF COMPLETE SURRENDER TO A FORCE GREATER THAN OURSELVES. THIS EXPERIENCE CAN BE SURPRISING, COMPELLING, AND BLISSFUL. AND IT APPEARS TO BE COMPLETELY OUT OF OUR CONTROL. WE CANNOT MAKE IT HAPPEN. WE CAN ONLY LET IT HAPPEN.

—— STEPHEN COPE

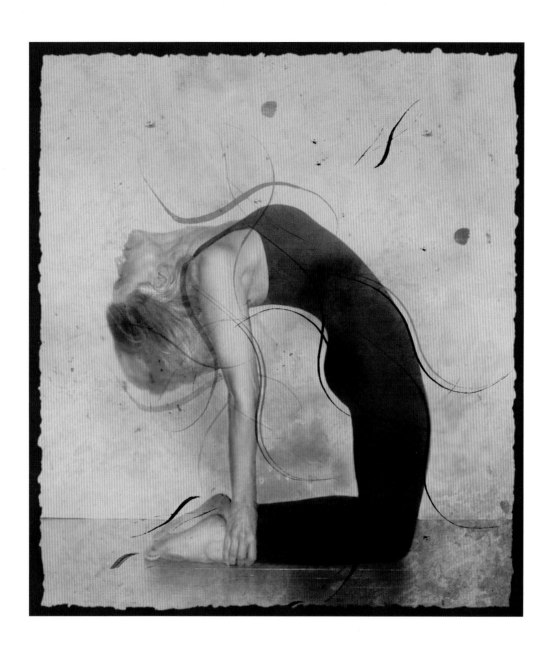

Camel Posture: Ustrasana

ONCE WE ACTUALLY BEGIN THIS YOGA PRACTICE AND START TO PAY ATTENTION A LITTLE MORE CLOSELY, WE BEGIN TO NOTICE HOW MUCH OF THE TIME WE ARE NOT PAYING ATTENTION AND HOW MUCH OF OUR LIFE PASSES US BY IN UNAWARENESS.

———— BERYL BENDER BIRCH

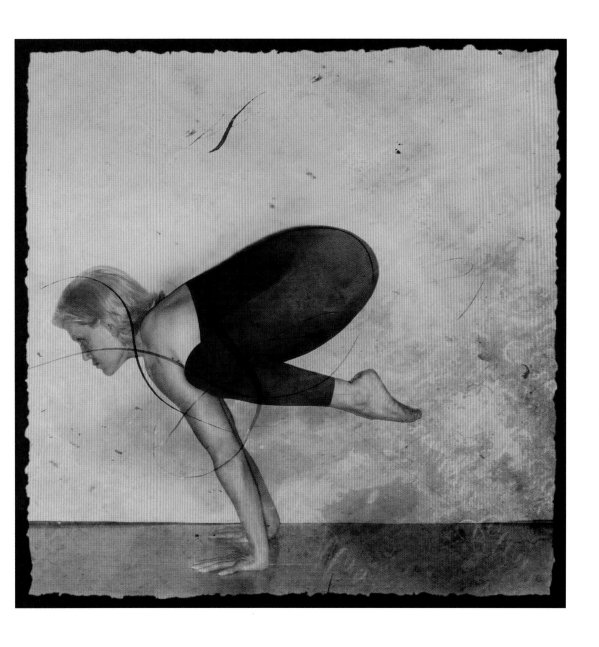

Crane Posture: Bakasana

ONE OF THE BASIC REASONS MANY PEOPLE TAKE UP YOGA IS TO CHANGE SOMETHING ABOUT THEMSELVES: TO BE ABLE TO THINK MORE CLEARLY, TO FEEL BETTER, AND TO BE ABLE TO ACT BETTER TODAY THAN THEY DID YESTERDAY IN ALL AREAS OF LIFE. IN THESE ENDEAVORS YOGA CAN BE OF GREAT HELP, AND IT REQUIRES NO PREREQUISITES THAT MUST BE FULFILLED BEFORE WE SET OUT ON THIS PATH.

—— T. K. V. DESIKACHAR

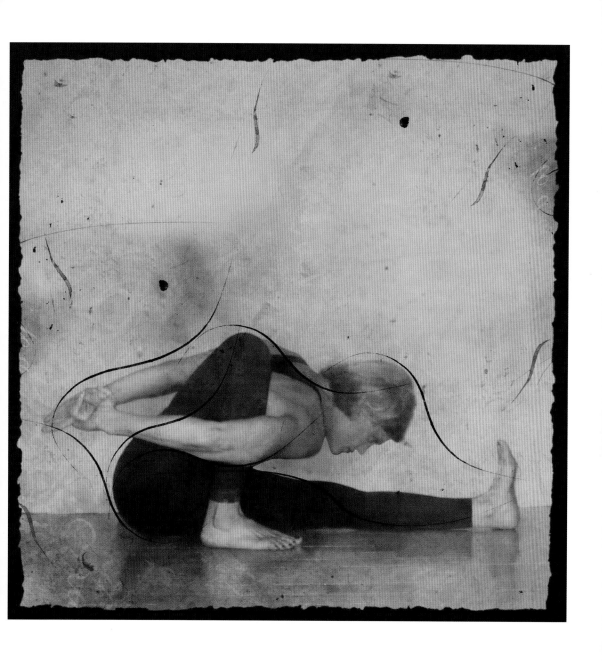

Dedicated to Marichi: Marichyasana A

THE BRAIN IS THE HARDEST
PART OF THE BODY TO ADJUST
IN ASANAS.

—— B. K. S. IYENGAR

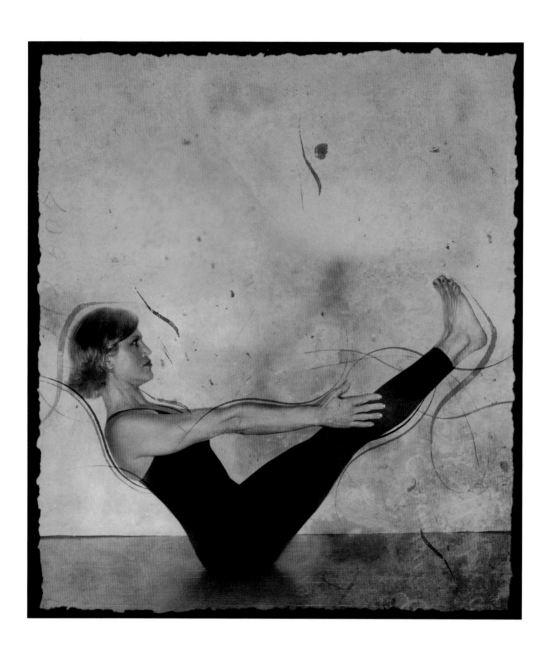

Boat Pose: Navasana

Y

OUR BODY MUST BE
DISCIPLINED LIKE A CHILD,
CALMLY BUT FORCEFULLY.
YOU ARE, IN FACT,
RE-EDUCATING YOUR BODY, AND
AS THE VARIOUS AREAS ARE
CONVINCED THAT YOU ARE
SERIOUS (JUST LIKE THE CHILD),
THEY WILL BEGIN TO OBEY.

——— RICHARD HITTLEMAN

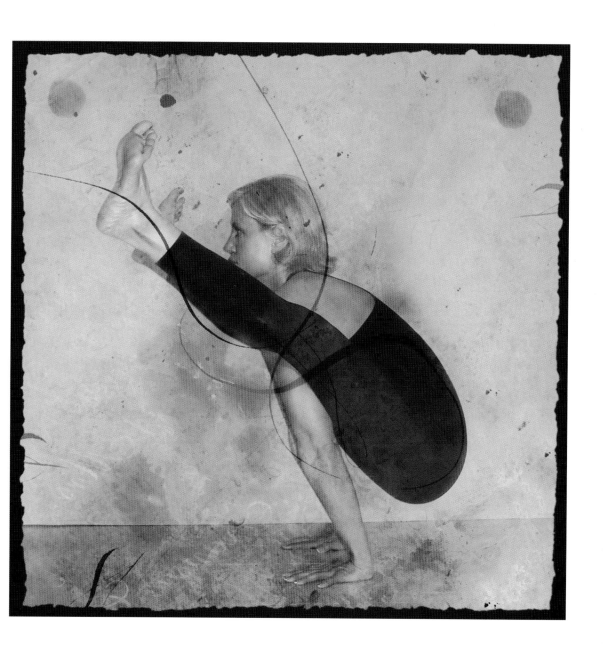

Firefly Posture: Tittibhasana

*P*EACE IS ALL AROUND US—IN THE
WORLD AND IN NATURE—AND
WITHIN US—IN OUR BODIES AND
OUR SPIRITS. ONCE WE LEARN TO
TOUCH THIS PEACE, WE WILL BE
HEALED AND TRANSFORMED. IT
IS NOT A MATTER OF FAITH; IT IS
A MATTER OF PRACTICE.

——— THICH NHAT HANH

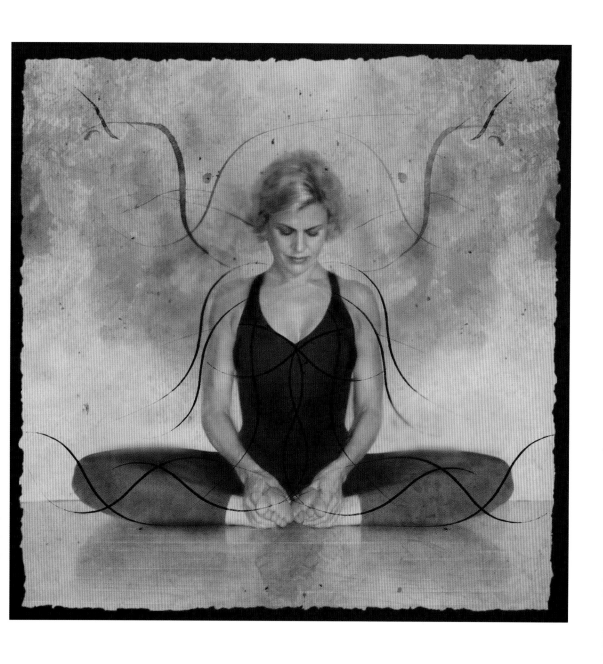

Bound Angle Posture: Baddha Konasana

CONCENTRATION IS LIKE A
DIAMOND, A BRILLIANT
FOCUSING OF OUR ENERGY,
INTELLIGENCE, AND SENSITIVITY.
WHEN WE CONCENTRATE FULLY,
THE LIGHT OF OUR ABILITIES
SHINES FORTH IN MANY COLORS,
RADIATING THROUGH ALL THAT
WE DO. OUR ENERGY GAINS A
MOMENTUM AND CLARITY THAT
ALLOWS US TO PERFORM EACH
TASK QUICKLY AND WITH EASE,
AND WE RESPOND TO THE
CHALLENGES WORK OFFERS WITH
PLEASURE AND ENTHUSIASM.

——— TARTHANG TULKU

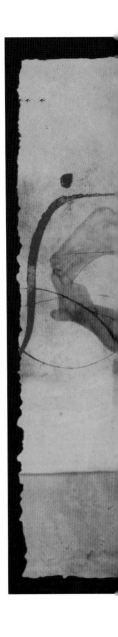

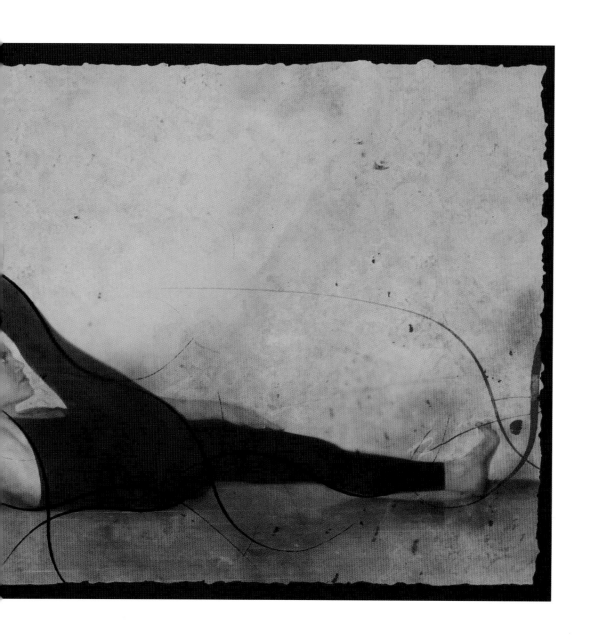

Sleeping Big Toe Posture: Supta Padangusthasana A

E

VERY BREATH CAN BE A
PRACTICE. WITH THE
INHALATION, IMAGINE DRAWING
IN PURE, CLEANSING, RELAXING
ENERGIES. AND WITH EACH
EXHALATION, IMAGINE
EXPELLING ALL OBSTACLES,
STRESS, AND NEGATIVE
EMOTIONS.

———— TENZIN WANGYAL RINPOCHE

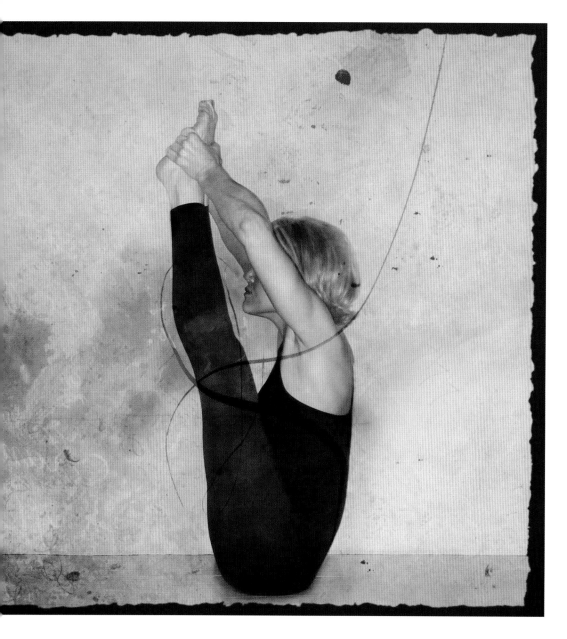

Upward Facing Intense West Stretch Pose:
Urdhva Mukha Paschimottanasana

THE POWER NEEDED IN YOGA IS THE POWER TO GO THROUGH EFFORT, DIFFICULTY, OR TROUBLE WITHOUT GETTING FATIGUED, DEPRESSED, DISCOURAGED, OR IMPATIENT AND WITHOUT BREAKING OFF THE EFFORT OR GIVING UP ONE'S AIM OR RESOLUTION. A QUIET, VIGILANT, BUT UNDISTRESSED PERSISTENCE IS THE BEST WAY TO GET YOGIC PRACTICE DONE.

———— SRI AUROBINDO

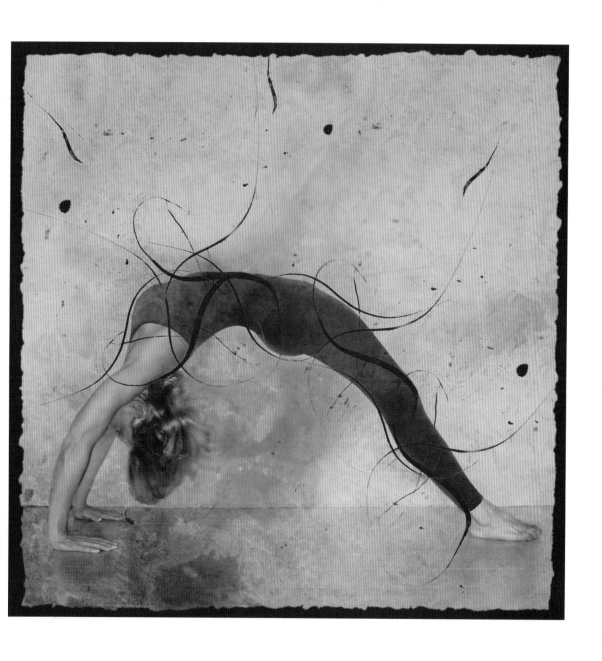

Wheel Posture: Urdhva Dhanurasana

*I*F YOU MAKE UP YOUR MIND
TO FIND JOY WITHIN YOURSELF,
SOONER OR LATER YOU SHALL
FIND IT.

—— PARAMAHANSA YOGANANDA

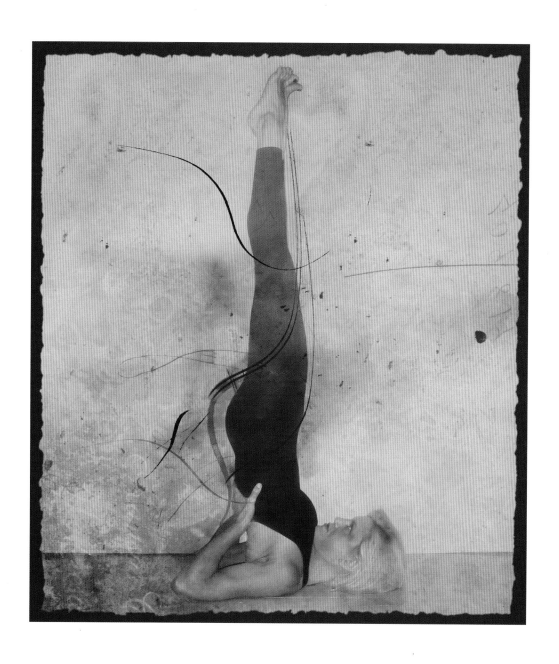

Shoulder Stand: Salamba Sarvangasana

*Y*OGA'S MESSAGES—RELAX, LET GO,
BREATHE, REMEMBER WHO YOU
ARE—WILL BEGIN TO REPLACE
SOCIETY'S MESSAGES OF PUSH,
SHOVE, GET AHEAD, AND LOOK OUT
FOR NUMBER ONE.

——— VICTORIA MORAN

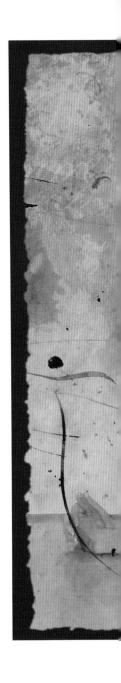

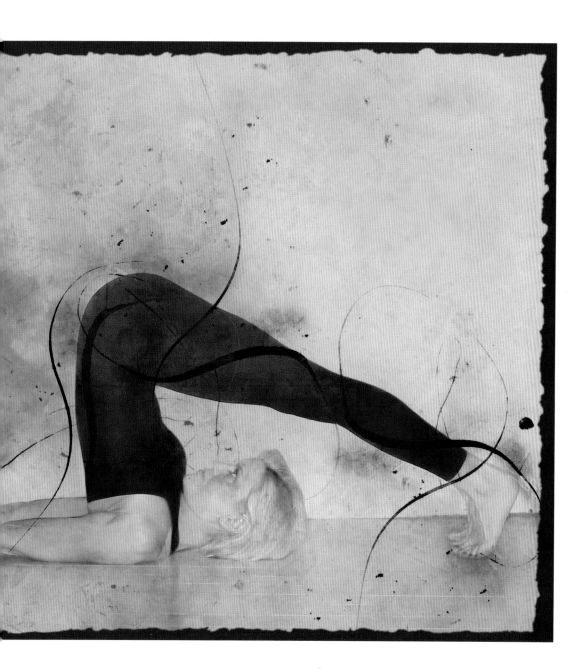

Plow Posture: Halasana

WHOLENESS IS PRECEDED BY FAITH, ENERGY, MINDFULNESS, UNION, AND AWARENESS.

———— YOGA SUTRA 1:20

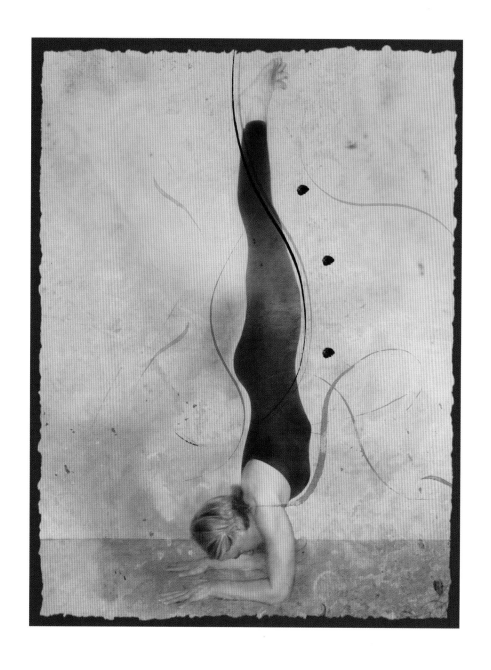

Feather of the Peacock: Pincha Mayurasana

THE ULTIMATE ATTAINMENT IS ALREADY OURS, BUT THE EXPERIENCE OF IT COMES TO US ONLY WHEN WE ARE IN A STATE OF COMPLETE SURRENDER. IN THIS CASE, "SURRENDER" MEANS THE SURRENDER OF EVERYTHING—EVERY EFFORT, DESIRE, THOUGHT OF ATTAINMENT, OR INDEED, ANYTHING THAT REPRESENTS THE THOUGHT OF ANY *other*—AS WE BECOME CENTERED, INSTEAD. THE PERSON WHO IS ABLE TO DO THIS BECOMES A FOUNTAIN OF CONSCIOUSNESS.

———— SWAMI CHETANANANDA

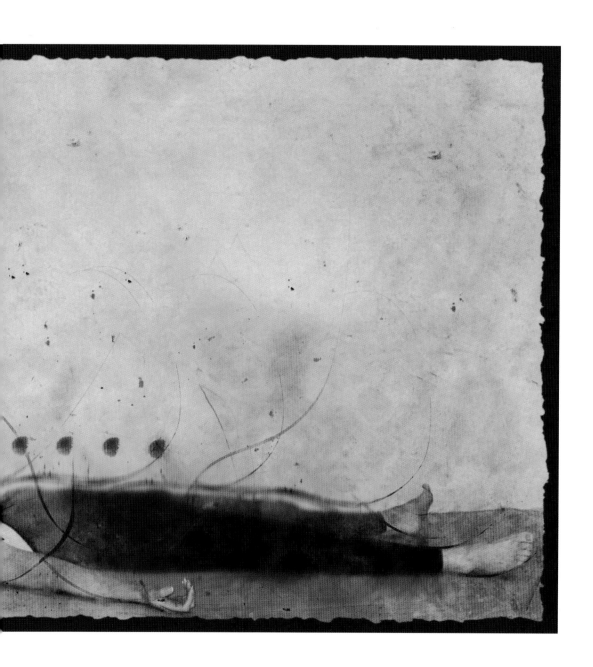

Corpse Pose: Savasana

Afterward

By Max Strom

Let us remember that the asanas are tools to rebuild ourselves. The goal is not to tie ourselves in knots, because we're already tied in knots. The aim is to untie the knots in our heart. The aim is to untie with the ultimate, loving, and peaceful power of the universe.

Namaste,

Max Strom

(Editor's note: Max Strom is an author, yoga instructor, and director of Sacred Movement Yoga in Venice, California.)

Acknowledgments

My gratitude to the following people for their support, help, and patience: Helen Ravenhill, Gretchen Robinson, Craig Neuman, Christine Dinyer, Dorothy O'Brien, Carolyn Howard-Johnson, Max Strom, Mark Blanchard, Genevieve and Keith Crosslin, Kathleen Kastner, Courtney Sullivan, John Carroll, and Ai Osada.

Please visit: www.effortandsurrender.com

About the Artist

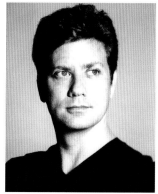

PHOTO BY KENNY JOHNSON

ERIC DINYER IS AN ILLUSTRATOR AND A DEDICATED YOGA PRACTITIONER. DINYER RECEIVED HIS B.F.A. FROM WASHINGTON UNIVERSITY IN ST. LOUIS, MISSOURI, AND HIS M.F.A. FROM THE SCHOOL OF VISUAL ARTS IN NEW YORK CITY, NEW YORK.

HE CURRENTLY LIVES IN THE MIDWEST WITH HIS WIFE, CHRISTINE, AND THEIR TWO SONS.

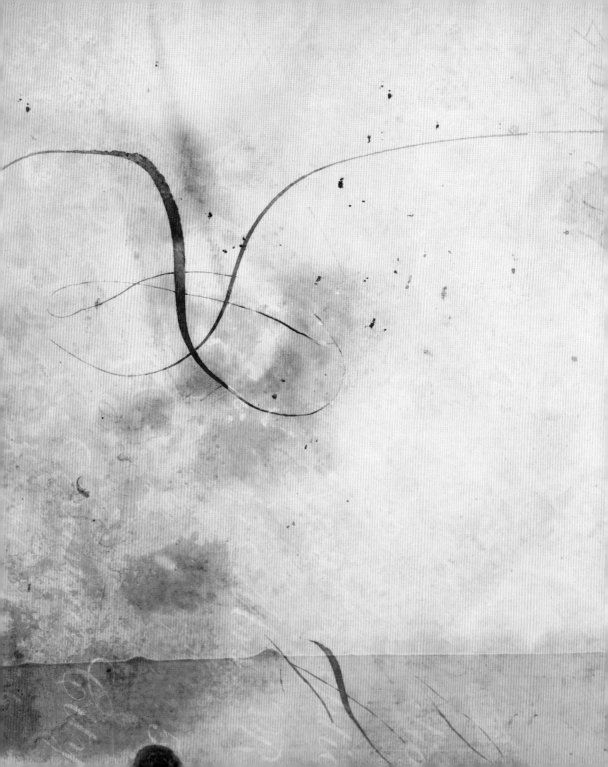

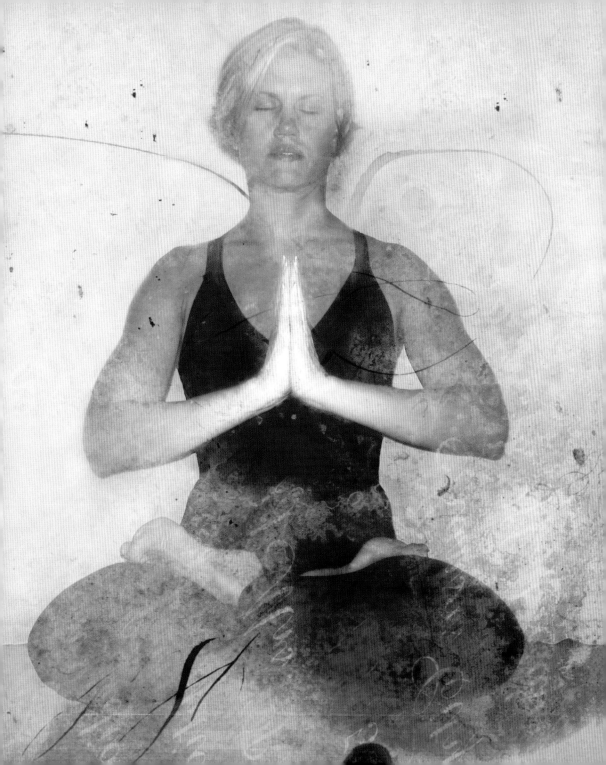

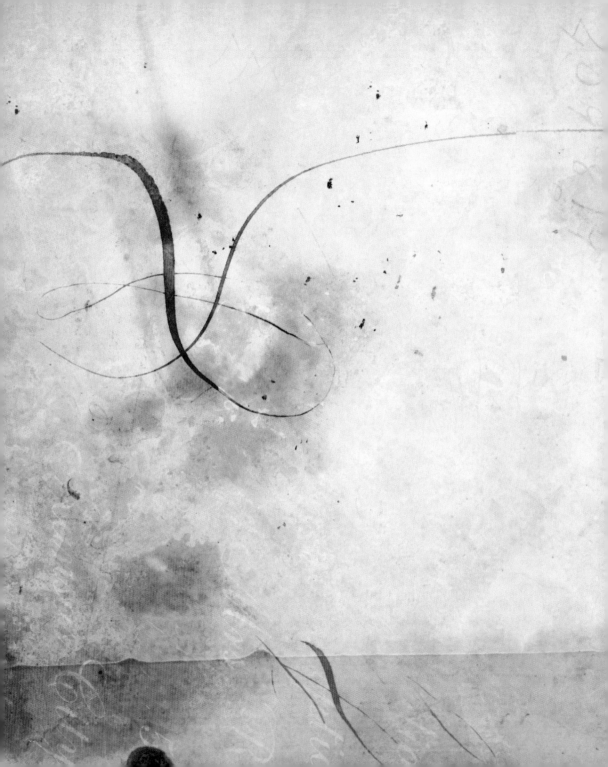